UnF**k Your Health

(Revised)

In his revised book "UnF**k Your Health" he not only gives up many guarded secrets in the medical, health, fitness and nutrition industry, but he added a new chapter dealing with his personal experience dealing with Covid, ...TWICE!

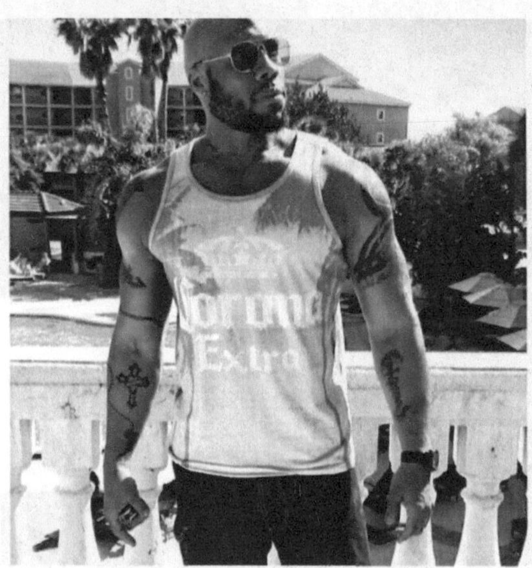

Originally from Boston, Massachusetts,

B. Rich Scott, Ordained Fitness Minister, knows firsthand what it takes to transform and improve the quality of your life. By utilizing the skills acquired and taught over the years. He worked for GNC over the span of 10 years and learned the game and created his own nutritional supplement brand. Combine that with over 20 years of training, coaching & competitive bodybuilding, B Rich lives his most passionate cause on a daily basis by assisting others in achieving their own body goals.

B Rich Scott offers a variety of services promoting the holistic wellbeing of mind, body and spirit including but not limited to Health & Fitness Coaching & Motivational Speaking. And explains how mentally being healthy placed a huge part in getting over it. B Rich can be found online at BRichScott.com and on Instagram.com/BRichScott.

Learn more about the “UnF**k Your Life” series: UnF**k Your Health An introductory guide to holistic healing for health & fitness. UnF**k Your Health gives a raw, uncut

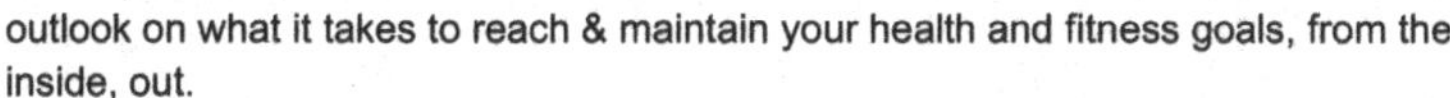
outlook on what it takes to reach & maintain your health and fitness goals, from the inside, out.

UnF**k Your Feelings comes as a timely, much needed perspective on the emotional responsibility of love & relationships. This title dives deep into the workings of emotions, along with the nature of men and women and how we respectively process shared experiences differently, while giving us the tools needed to play the "dating game" effectively through 'smart work' rather than hard work.

Ordering Information: Quantity sales. Special discounts are available on quantity purchases by email address above. Orders by U.S. trade bookstores and wholesalers.

Please contact 526 Publishing: Tel: (617) 905-3779; or visit www.brichscott.com.

Printed in the United States of America

Forewarning- Adult Language and Extremely Strong Sexual Overtone

This is the introduction to my new book series titled: UnF**k Your Life. I have to stress this here and often throughout the book. My writing style is very unconventional and may take some time to adjust to, but it will not be difficult to follow along. I wanted any and everyone that knows how to read to be able to comprehend and take in the extremely important jewels of wisdom that I am dropping in this book. This book was actually fun to write and I have a feeling it will be more fun to read. It may have a few people in their feelings at times, but fuck your feelings. Trust me, you need to know what you need to know and I'm telling it.

What Is The Reason For This Book?

To those who really know me, I write how I talk, so you will have to take the traditional way of reading (or how one writes) out of the equation and just pretend I'm talking to you. So this book will go ALL OVER THE PLACE. Don't worry, it's supposed to, but it will always come back to make a point. As you read, try to have an open mind, because it will be easier for you to digest. In doing so, I hope to keep you engaged, stimulated, educated, inspired and quite possibly aroused. So be prepared for that off the jump. Let me be clear, there are numerous ways one can achieve a good looking body, but this book is about more than just the physical. Much more!

In this book, I will go into how food and exercise not only affect the types of romantic and emotional relationships people have with one another but also how it affects the spirit, the mind, and the body. Hopefully, through understanding this paradigm, you will have the tools to establish a discipline that will help you transcend towards a holistic approach to nutrition if you choose to. I'm going to give you a completely different perspective on how foods affect one's life. My vast knowledge and wisdom in this arena are way too complex to put down in just this one book, especially one of this length, but I wanted to create a quick read for some of my fans, past lovers and future clients, to be able to refer to for the time being. I will have other projects and materials regarding health, relationships, astrology, universal laws and spiritual laws that will be coming down the Mass pike in the near future.

With that being said, this will be the most peculiar take on health and fitness that you will ever have the pleasure to read...and boy, if you thought the original was a piece of work, wait until you get a load of what I have in the revised version. I do not think anyone has yet to put it together quite in this way. Blame it on my Gemini dual brain capacity. Hopefully, this will not only be informative, but extremely entertaining and provocative as well. How can a nutrition book be provocative and seductive? Oh! Did I say seductive? Guess we'll just have to find out together. Enjoy and learn something you may not have known or watch as I place a new spin on something you may already know.

He Fked Up Breakfast for Me**

How many people understand what breakfast means? Such a simple question, but the answer may be loaded with such ignorance. Why do some people feel that cereal, eggs, bacon, and pancakes are breakfast foods? Some people are so indoctrinated with societal programming that they may physically get sick if they eat anything other than "breakfast" foods for breakfast. I have heard people say foods like pizza or pasta are too heavy for their stomachs. Yet, foods like pancakes, muffins, and donuts, which are traditionally breakfast foods, are some of the most dense and heaviest foods to eat any time of day, if we're going to be honest.

Most people have been programmed through marketing and repetition to create an unnatural and unreal "reality" that has real potentially dangerous consequences. So what does breakfast mean? I mean literally, what does the word breakfast mean? I'll wait...

Many people do not realize that the word "breakfast" is actually two separate words, BREAK and FAST. "Fast" or fasting is the willing abstinence or reduction of some, or all food, drink, or both, for a period of time. "An absolute fast or 'dry fasting' is normally defined as abstinence from all food and liquid for a defined period." -per Wikipedia. Some people fast for religious reasons, spiritual reasons, training reasons and a variety of other reasons. But no matter the reason, EVERYONE does a fast in some shape, form or fashion.

Most do it unconsciously, like when they go to sleep. The length of time is also very important when we are talking about *consciously* fasting. Fasting helps with the spirit and it is another great tool to have in your bag to utilize. The act of eating is what "breaks" a fast. And contrary to what many have been conditioned to believe, breakfast does not have a "time" of day associated with it. If I go to bed at 8 am then wake up at 4 pm... And then decide to eat, my body does not know what time of the day it is, it just knows that it needs calories. And once my body has taken in those calories, I have broken my fast. Even something as simple as juice can break a fast. It's all about the calories being consumed.

Sidebar: Millions of people drink coffee for breakfast. A lot of people say that they like coffee, but this is not necessarily true. What most people like is the caffeine in the coffee. Want to see how true this statement is? Ask the next caffeinated coffee drinker you meet why don't they get the decaffeinated version, many will look at you like you are crazy. Caffeine is a very powerful drug, now put that together with the most powerful drug in the world; sugar, you may be hooked for life.

Here is the problem; caffeine is highly addictive and it can obstruct the activity of adenosine, a neurotransmitter that affects almost every bodily function. The main job of adenosine is to make us tired or sleepy, caffeine blocks the absorption of adenosine; this keeps us from feeling fatigued. Not really a good thing when it is abused by people. Because caffeine is not illegal, many think that it is safe. *It is really not*. Did you know that if a person over 150 lbs was to snort 5 grams of cocaine, the person may get high as fuck, but most likely will not overdose and die? But what if I told you, that if you were to measure the same 5 grams, but replace the word cocaine with *caffeine*, you would overdose and most likely die of a heart attack.

Look how we started that off… pretty good, right? Well, we 'bout to blast the fuck off...

Buckle up!

What Is It About Me?

I've been a personal trainer for the past 12 years, but more importantly than that, I have been well educated in nutrition for even longer. I did not just stumble into this lifestyle; this lifestyle has always been with me. I did not know what this "feeling" was in regards to being healthy, nor did I know anything about what it meant to be "healthy", but I always knew as a young boy, that I wanted to be strong and to look strong. I did not know how I knew at the time, but I intuitively felt that food was a way to help shape that reality.

When most children look at superheroes, they don't look at Superman, Batman, or Spiderman and think to themselves about food or exercise. Consciously, they know that in many cases these superheroes got their "powers" from some kind of strange happenstance or they were born with it... well, except for Popeye, spinach was his claim to fame.

Sidebar: Did you know that Popeye was a whole propaganda game just so that people could eat more spinach? Here is some information about Popeye and Spinach that many were gushing over back in the day. "Popeye, with his odd accent and improbable forearms, used spinach to great effect, a sort of anti-Kryptonite. It gave him his strength, and perhaps his distinctive speaking style. But why did Popeye eat so much spinach? What was the reason for his obsession with such strange food? The truth begins more than fifty years earlier. Back in 1870, Erich von Wolf, a German chemist, examined the amount of iron within spinach, among many other green vegetables. In recording his findings, von Wolf accidentally misplaced a decimal point when transcribing data from his notebook, changing the iron content in spinach by an order of magnitude. While there are actually only 3.5 milligrams of iron in a 100-gram serving of spinach, the accepted fact became *35 milligrams*.

To put this in perspective, if the calculation were correct each 100-gram serving would be like eating a small piece of a paper clip. Once this incorrect number was printed, spinach's nutritional value became legendary. So when Popeye was created, studio executives recommended he eat spinach for his strength, due to its vaunted health properties. Apparently Popeye helped increase American consumption of spinach by a third! This error was eventually corrected in 1937 when someone rechecked the numbers. But the damage had been done. It spread and spread, and only recently has gone by the wayside, no doubt helped by Popeye's relative obscurity today. But the error was so widespread that the British Medical Journal published an article discussing this spinach incident in 1981, trying its best to finally debunk the issue."
-https://www.brainpickings.org/2013/07/02/spinach-popeye-error-halflife-of-facts/

In watching these fictional heroes do powerful things, it makes a young child want to try to do those powerful things as well. He or she quickly realizes that they need some strength to even be able to do a fraction of physical activity. So the first thing that usually comes to mind at a young age for most kids, if you want to be strong, working out will help you become a superhero. Food is generally not something most adults even really comprehend when it comes to strength, or how one uses it to change the composition of their body, so think about how unlikely it is for a child to equate food to strength or to develop muscles in the body.

Somewhere deep down inside my core, I knew the food that I was consuming was going to be a major part of my superpowers. I was around 7 years old and had sat at the table preparing for lunch. Hot dogs and Ramen noodles. This was one of my favorite meals. At that age in my life, the flavorful seasoned noodles, mixed with the savory blend of sensations from the ketchup and mustard on the fork from my hot dog, was an exquisite and complementary combination of taste. It was exciting to my young palate. However, this particular day was different. I noticed something that I had never really paid attention to.

I took a closer look at the noodles on my plate and noticed that they were extremely oily. This was odd to me, considering that these noodles came directly out of boiling water. Oily though? How could this be? My conscious mind was at work. I had watched spaghetti plenty of times coming out of boiling water to be sticky and almost dry, but not oily. So I wanted to know why these noodles had been so greasy. I looked at the package and started reading the ingredients.

This was something that I used to do when I would sit down for breakfast and read the cereal box cover to cover. Usually, there would be some kind of fun game in the back for kids to play. After I was done with the game, I would read the nutritional panel for the products that actually had them labeled on the boxes back then.

Sidebar: Back in the day, food industries were not required to print nutritional facts on the labels of the food we eat....and to be quite frank, even in 2021 we still can't be sure of the true contents in what we consume. Can we really believe that the calories, fats, carbohydrates, and proteins have the actual numbers that they are said to contain? Just know that a lot of companies "eyeball" or wing it with these nutritional "facts."

Just placing another tool in your tool kit.

I got quite familiar with different ingredients and started to pay close attention to anything regarding nutrition, foods, muscle, exercise, and fat in the news. As I looked over this package of Ramen noodles, I saw the word "partially hydrogenated oil" as the main ingredient, but at the time I had no idea what that was, although it always stuck in my mind.

Meanwhile, I continued to eat the delicious noodles. In my pre-teen years, I started watching WWF wrestling. I could not wait until Saturday morning at 11 a.m. to tune in to the Superstars of Wrestling. I admired the muscles and athletic frames and wanted to get my body in shape like the superheroes on my TV screen. I thought to myself, I'll get like that one day. That was the first time that I can actually remember exercising. I had found a gold plastic dumbbell in my mother's room that weighed about 8 lbs. It was filled concrete and sand of some kind.

My mother didn't like me going into her room taking things out and playing with them, but in my mind, this was no play. I was serious about putting on some muscle even though I had no idea what that really meant and how to actually do it. I would stand in my room in front of my small black and white television while wrestling was on and started doing curls and push-ups through the whole one-hour program. (Look at the word I just used "program"...pay attention)

I would take breaks during commercials. From that point on, I started doing more and more reading regarding food and exercise.

I read every magazine and watched every news clip or article on health-related things. I was determined to get my body like one of those men that I saw on my TV screen and I was determined to be just as strong. This is where my fascination with all things regarding health would begin.

What Does Healthy Mean?

Most people have no clue what healthy really is or what healthy really means. We may look at a person and see that they may have some, or a lot of muscles, and confuse that "nice-looking body" that appeals to the eyes visually, for a person being healthy internally. In fact, in a lot of cases, nothing can be further from the truth. Let's take a further look into this.

We all know someone in the past or present who could eat whatever they wanted on God's green earth and not only did they not gain a pound, but their body was in exceptional shape visually. But what some of you do not realize, is that the insides of their bodies, as far as the blood, enzymes, bacteria and hormone levels were not healthy and pretty soon would start to reflect externally in just a few short years. And even if the body still appeared to be healthy, blood and lab work can tell a different story.

There was a book that came out in 2005 called, "Natural Cures the "Truth" They Do Not Want You to Know", by Kevin Trudeau. That book took a lot of ignorance and bliss out of my world regarding food and what I considered healthy at the time and put a crash course of harsh truths to my sense of conventional reality. There was a new stage being set and that stage was ushering in a new kind of food called genetically modified organisms (GMOs). At first, this was something that was spun as being healthy and good for you, but Kevin broke that all the way down in his book on why it was not. Along with that, he went into exposing a lot of the shady practices of hiding stuff in the labeling of foods, and obviously dangerous feat.

This book was so controversial and so damaging on exposing the FDA, that the book was banned at one point. Now there are a large group of people that completely disagree with a lot of things he writes in the book regarding cures on AIDS, cancer, amongst other things, but I will say this, that book single-handedly changed how I looked at the FDA and the food industry. It's shameful and immoral how these commercials and companies are pushing these false "healthy" labeled products to the consumer.

But fuck morality and your health. "Gimme the loot, Gimme the loot" One of the biggest fads initially for a health-conscious lifestyle was the consumption of soy milk. In the mid 1980s it was introduced as a healthier alternative to cow's milk, along with a whole host of additional attractive benefits. Cutting fat was the wave back then, and soy milk consisted of almost half the fat of regular milk. That was enough to get the ball rolling. After a while, it was showing up everywhere. Coincidentally, do you know what else started to pop up years later at a more rapid pace? Breast cancer!

When you start looking at the properties and biology of food, you only then start to really understand how it affects your properties and biology of yourself on the inside. When you think about working out, one usually thinks in terms of physical activity, in the vain of exercise, which usually includes some sort of aerobic activity or strength training... maybe both. This in itself is not enough for you to get full cooperation from the body to be the best version of itself.

There is an old saying that goes "You can't outrun a bad diet", which in layman's terms means, no matter how much you work out physically if your diet is not good, the results will be minimal at best.

I didn't realize how important this was until, I started to train in order to not only be stronger, but also to change the way my physique was shaped. Talking about training, in which the way the body, chemically and physically can be changed drastically by the way you put certain calories together. It is sometimes like trying to explain quantum physics of the universe to someone, which sometimes may be a lot easier to understand. We have a whole industry of health and medical professionals that can't seem to get this nutrition thing right...or so it appears.

What Do Food And Drugs Have To Do With One Another?

Why is it that food has been scientifically proven to change your hormones, but is not labeled as a drug? Well in order to answer that question, you would first have to believe that the FDA, your doctors and nutrition "experts" actually want you to be healthy. And if you do happen to believe that, that's part of the main issue millions of Americans have today. They believe the fucking lie!

Let's start with some basic fundamentals, so that we can at a minimum, all be at a basic understanding of how food works and the biochemistry, numbers, and profiles behind it. The FDA classifies a drug as "A substance recognized by an official pharmacopeia or formulary. A substance intended for use in the diagnosis, cure, mitigation, treatment, or prevention of disease. A substance (other than food) intended to affect the structure or any function of the body."

A drug is any substance that causes a change in an organism's physiology or psychology when consumed. Drugs are typically distinguished from food and substances that provide nutritional support. Hmm, that is quite an interesting definition for what a drug is. But here is the really interesting part of that... Did you know that in order to get something classified as a drug it needs a patent? And this can cost millions of dollars!

Also, if you made a claim that a food blend that you put together can cure a disease, you could be fined a lot of money...I mean, unless you were able to get a patent for that food blend. I have my own nutritional supplement brand, *B. Rich Wellness* and I personally have taken MANY foods and my own supplements that have (I cannot say the,"C" word) but it rhymes with *'PURED'* people of certain ailments. You know it's some funny business going on when you don't even have the freedom to publish them in a book without the risk of being a target.

Imagine that. I will touch back on this at a later point.

I did not want this to be a typical boring nutrition and fitness book, but there are some things that you must know in order to understand the game as I continue to drop it.

What Is A Calorie?

A calorie is a unit of energy. In nutrition, calories refer to the energy people get from the food and drink they consume, and the energy they use in physical activity.

What Are Macronutrients? In order for your body to perform on any level, it needs a source of energy. That energy comes in the form of calories. Calories are broken down into 4 categories.

The four principal classes of calories or macronutrients are carbohydrates, protein, lipids and alcohol.

Macronutrients are a class of chemical compounds people consume in the largest quantities which provide people with the bulk of energy.

To keep it simple and break this down even further, calories come in the form of 3 numbers.

(9, 4 and 7) And here is where the MOST important part of the game, as far as body composition is concerned.

One gram of fat = 9 calories One gram of alcohol (which is sugar) =7 calories One gram of carbohydrate = 4 calories One gram of protein = 4 calories These numbers are the most important numbers that you need to know because these are the building blocks and foundation on how you put total calories together and the master key on how you design your calorie intake for gains or loss.

Once you are able to learn and excel at this you have yet another very important and handy tool in your toolbox. That's my word. Let's take a mental and inspirational break here. I want to take the time here to express how extremely important discipline is in this journey that you are about to forego, this is part of the foundation as well. Discipline will be needed throughout. I will discuss how changing the food you consume will change and enhance your discipline shortly, but first let's unpack this calorie equation a little bit further.

I always say, "Calories are not created equal." It sounds simple to those that know and understand this, but most do not truly understand this concept. As I stated before, I do not want this to be overly complicated, so I will give this simple example.

Let's say I had a friend who was my same height, but was a little bit smaller in frame, but wanted to get to my size and build. I am 6'0", 240 lbs. Let's say that in order to maintain my frame and size, I needed 3,500 calories a day. My friend asks me about my calorie intake. He goes and consumes 3,500 calories a day for the next month, but most of his calories are coming in the form of fats and carbs and from a little bit of alcohol. I see him a month later and look at him. I can tell he has obviously gained some size, but a lot of it is in the form of body fat and not actually healthy muscle tissue.

He is now upset and frustrated that he undertook this 3,500 calorie a day challenge, but still does not look like me. Although this is a hypothetical example, this type of thing happens ALL THE TIME when it comes to people spinning their wheels when it comes to the "calorie boogeyman". You hear about dropping calories, increasing calories, burning calories. Calories! Calories! Calories! And as much information that is out there, still, most seem to get this all wrong. Part of the problem with my "friend" in the example above, was that he, unfortunately, thought all calories were the same.

He did not understand how important what source(s) he was actually getting his calories from in order to make up that 3,500 calorie goal. If he would have asked me, I would have told him to put more of his calorie bulk in the form of lean protein and complex carbs, but this is also something that can be tricky because what most experts don't tell you, or even take into account, is that your energy output will drastically determine how much calories you may need for a specific goal.

Also, it is important to understand how emotional issues can play a part in how your calories are being "burned" or used. Some carbs are very powerful when it comes to helping some people deal with minor depression and/or emotional issues. Some carbs help to make new serotonin.

Serotonin makes us feel calmer and helps us relax. So what can potentially happen if a person is not privy to how this affects your chemistry and biology, a person will eat the carb to feel good and the more they consume, the better they feel. Sometimes in this space of feeling so good, they completely forgo any discipline with the diet and instead keep chasing after this "high" in order to keep the serotonin coming in. The body is slowly starting to become immune to the levels currently being taken in, which send a signal to the brain (which loves the serotonin), that it needs more, so you consume more to keep your hormone levels regulated. Carbohydrates spike insulin levels, however, if you were to eliminate carbs and stick to a lean protein and moderate fat diet, some people can avoid it, I'm not supposed to say it, because there is no "cure" for diabetes... But the information is out there. Go figure. Research the KETO diet for more information on that, the history behind it is quite interesting.

But let's get back to business… Because I have been training for many years, I have learned my body and have unlocked the mysteries and science of food so I can transform my body on a whim very easily. The combination of food and exercise are no longer the hardest part once you are this deep in, it is the discipline that takes most of the bulk here. Back when my grandparents were growing up, the food was just different. We all hear that, but many have no clue how important that is or even why it is important.

Before the late 80s and 90s, food had more of their actual food profiles that they are supposed to have in them currently. If one orange was supposed to contain 100% of vitamin C, it was fair to say that it did back then. Today? Not so much. You would be lucky to get half of that with the oranges you get today, and that's if you can even get a hold of a real orange.

Sidebar: Nutritional supplements are an extremely chaotic and confusing arena if you do not know how to navigate through it. Fortunately, I understood it well enough that I decided to open my own nutritional supplement company *B. Rich Wellness*, but that was not before the original copy of this book was printed in October of 2019.

Here is what I will say, the reason we ALL need some sort of supplementation is because all the nutrition from food you once did you are not getting anymore. Many companies, including mine, have found a way to profit by providing you an unnatural way to supplement your dietary needs with something that you should be getting naturally. (I am being very transparent here)

Now before you think that I'm trying to put down supplement companies (which I am not, ahem, *B. RICH WELLNESS*), just know that I have taken plenty of supplements and will continue to take supplements the rest of my life, because I see the value in SOME of them.

However, if I did not have to, trust me, I wouldn't. Unfortunately, many foods have no nutrition to levels they should have! I cannot emphasize that enough. (Well at least in the Western Hemisphere)The problem is that a lot of companies are giving you stuff that you really do not need. Giving you stuff that is not authentic. Giving you stuff that is not doing what they say it's supposed to do. And in "Bizarro World" this is a real thing, the companies that actually do give a good quality product that might actually help and do what it's supposed to, the FDA will ban it and have you depending on their dangerous prescription medications.

I can literally write a whole 200 page book on supplements, but I won't do it.

At least not at this time. When you have food that is in its proper form, food that the universe created in its perfection, it is in tune with the body and the human spirit, which connects mind and soul. We will get real deep into that soon because I can go from zero to 100 real quick with this information. The book I referenced earlier by Kevin Trudeau, A LOT of people were not ready for that kind of honesty and knowledge and many still aren't.

The foods that our grandparents ate were of better quality. My grandmother died at the age of 90, but her physical strength and blood work up to her mid-80s were immaculate. I knew a lot of men in their late 60's and 70's when I was a teenager and some of those men were in better shape than some of the 30 and 40-yearold men today. I contribute a huge amount of that to the food, but there are also other factors that indirectly relate to the food as far as I'm concerned. When we see how important testosterone levels are in men, we see where a whole society can take a left turn when these levels are unbalanced.

Male Hormonal Levels

This was a taboo topic at one point, but because of such widespread impotency, obese men (some in the shape of women), as well as a surge of emotionally unstable men, there was eventually going to be some kind of backlash and it has been steadily building momentum throughout that past few decades. I know what I am about to say will turn away a huge segment of readers, but "Oh, Fckn' well!" You cannot manipulate Mother Nature and the Laws of the Universe and think that there will not be consequences.

Here is my personal opinion in which I will explain biologically. Again, you may not agree, but the truth is the truth. This is not MY truth. *It's biology.*

There has been a rise in homosexuality because food is being manipulated. Bet I got ya attention now! Let's dissect this.

We know that both males and females have two specific hormones that determine and make each who they are. Men primarily have testosterone and women primarily have estrogen. We understand that each has some of the other hormones in them as well, but to a lesser degree, NATURALLY. Before we can jump to the full conclusion, we first have to establish certain truths. To start, we know that men have certain attributes that they possess because they are male, period. Usually, this will include more muscle mass or the capacity to gain muscle quicker, can grow facial hair, deeper voice, usually taller, and usually attracted to women by the nature of energy.

Masculine energy will be attracted to its opposite, feminine energy. I have to say this as a disclaimer because there are exceptions to every rule, but some people wish to be contrary just to be so I will say "generally speaking" this is usually the case to C.M.A. Do we all agree that it is a factual statement? Ok, let us go to my second statement. Again, GENERALLY SPEAKING, because of women's estrogenic properties, they usually will consist of a smaller frame, usually, be curvier, usually can develop breasts, have menstrual cycles, and usually are attracted to men by the nature of energy. Feminine energy will be attracted to its opposite.

Do we all agree that this is a factual statement? If you do not, research your biology books.

Let's continue. When we look at the two examples above, if we are being honest, if you stand a male and a female next to one another you should be able to see a difference (well at least there was definitely a time where you could clearly see the differences, but in this day and age not so much, which brings me to my point) What is the main difference between the two? Hmm, well let's see. They both have a head, a torso, arms, and legs...but the genitalia is different, right? And what determines that? The MAIN difference is one human is made up more of testosterone and the other human is made up more of estrogen.

Now that we got that out of the way, let me break down some other interesting things about both of these hormones. Let's not forget the female menstrual cycle. The reason why a woman is usually more soft-spoken, calmer and more emotional in her feelings than a man is because of that powerful hormone Estrogen. This is in fact, what makes her attracted to the opposite sex OR SOMETHING COMPARABLE TO THE RECEPTION OF HER ENERGY.... Follow me here.

If I know that by nature, a woman will be attracted to the opposite energy, For the purpose of procreation, the main reason why you have genitals in the first place) then by default, I can already figure out how to attract her to another HUMAN, no matter the gender if I can configure a way to reprogram her hormonal wiring. Are you with me so far?

In an earlier chapter, I explained how food can change your hormone levels and literally have your brain produce other hormones, do you think that science does not know this and this is all just one big coincidence that homosexuality is on the rise? We know for a fact that certain products like the soy they were promoting and pushing as a healthy alternative has been proven to raise estrogen levels, we know that certain over-the-counter drugs have hormones in them that increase and act like estrogen. We know that certain additives and preservatives not only block your pineal gland and calcify it, which I will go into later, but the plastic containers that hold your water have all been proven to leach BPAs in the water that mimics estrogen.

Want to go deeper down that rabbit hole? Of course, you do.

Many women put on cosmetics, like foundation, lipsticks, lip gloss, blush, perfumes, lotions, hair products that all contain powerful chemicals that actually increase their estrogenic hormone levels. This is important to understand before I go into my next example. When a baby is initially created, the fetus appears to be sexually indifferent, meaning that it neither appears to be a male or a female. Over the next five to six weeks, the fetus begins producing hormones that cause its sex organs to develop and form into either male or female organs. But if the baby, while still in the womb, has been determined to be a male child, and that woman continues to put products on her skin and in her body that is elevating her estrogen levels, it's actually raising that male baby's estrogen levels as well.

So if we know that the foods of today lack the nutritional value that our forefathers used to eat and that the food we consume now has been hijacked and replaced with hormones and chemicals to enhance estrogen levels, then what do you think the odds of a tiny little baby boy, who has zero to no testosterone in his body is going to be faced with as he gets older?

Probably a higher estrogenic profile, right? Do you think there just may be a possibility that he may start thinking like a girl? And if he starts to think like a girl, do you think that there just may be a possibility that he starts acting like a girl? And if that is the case, how long do you think it will be before he starts being attracted to what other humans with a higher level of estrogen are attracted to?

Just my thoughts. So as we talk about the male and the female, now would be a good time to transition into how foods can affect everything in our lives, especially, believe or not, our personal relationships. Again, this is not a traditional fitness book. And if you're still reading up to this point, good! We are going in. I am going to go places that most people not only will not go but do not understand.

Let's put a new word into the lexicon in regards to nutrition. That word is metaphysics.

What Is Metaphysics?

Metaphysical, Derived from the Greek word "Meta Physika" ("after the things of nature"); referring to an idea, doctrine, or posited reality outside of human sense perception ...in layman's terms, meaning "That shit crazy." In modern philosophical terminology, metaphysics refers to the studies of what cannot be reached through objective studies of material reality.

Why is this specific term of importance? Because sometimes science cannot explain all the things that happen or can be proven. When we look at things like manifestation and the ideology behind that, we understand most of this cannot tangibly be proven with a conventional scientific formula. However, those who understand the Laws of the Universe and the spiritual side of this know for a fact that tangible results can be produced from such unconventional methods. Part of this is, we have to understand that tangible and intangible realities are created by thoughts. Anything and everything that you currently have at your disposal was created in someone's mind.

If you look at conventional science, how can they draw that in an equation? I'll show you how. If we dissect that in simpler terms, those that fall in line with science, on either side, we can say that, if one creates something out of pure thought, then there is some kind of mental energy that you cannot see or touch, that created something that you can see or touch. This is called Intentional manifestation. If science can prove that we create tangible realities just by pure thought alone means that manifestation exists in the realm of conventional science.

Thoughts create your reality. The placebo effect is an example of metaphysics that is widely accepted within the scientific community. Here is an interesting article that I happen to read for research purposes on examples of metaphysics: "Studies have shown that thoughts alone can improve vision, fitness, and strength. The placebo effect, as observed with fake operations and sham drugs, for example, works because of the power of thought. Expectancies and learned associations have been shown to change brain chemistry and circuitry which results in real physiological and cognitive outcomes, such as less fatigue, lower immune system reaction, elevated hormone levels, and reduced anxiety."

This research gives credence for metaphysics to the non-believers and for those that may be on the fence about where I'm going next with the game.

Women, a Party in Your Mouth can be directly Associated with a Party in ya P*ssy!

Let me paint you a picture. A woman is out dancing with her girls on a Saturday night. The weather is lovely and she is looking just as beautiful as the weather feels. She has many eyes and admirers watching her. She feels awesome. Her estrogenic levels are on high and her pheromones are attracting the opposite sex to her even more because of the elevated estrogen. She catches an attractive male at the bar. He comes over and says, "Hi". Her natural energy is receptive and she says hello back as she smiles with her eyes. He offers to buy her a drink. She accepts. She drinks her poison as the two of them begin to talk. As the alcohol starts to work its way through her body, it starts to somewhat change the biochemistry that regulates certain hormones and blood levels.

She starts to feel her temperature rise because the sugar from the alcohol has spiked her estrogen level and her body has to raise the blood pressure slightly to keep up with the other bioengineering faculties. Even a slight increase of 1 or 2 points, in either direction regarding blood pressure, can be felt to a person who is really in tune with their body. The conversation is great. He offers to buy her another drink, she accepts. Raspberry-Vanilla Martini. She starts to feel more relaxed in this man's presence, who she does not know, but something in her brain is telling her that this feels right. That's the serotonin again making another guest appearance. The job of that hormone is to calm you down. Remember alcohol is nothing but simple sugar. And remember simple carbs convert into simple sugar and therefore have the same effects as that cookie we spoke of earlier.

Her defense levels are now down and because of this; she does not realize the body language cues that she is giving off to this guy, who she does not know. And what she also does not know, is that this guy is pretty good at understanding food bioengineering and is going to manipulate her body to bend to his desire. He starts to watch her more closely as she takes her next sip. Her body language was more reserved initially, but he is watching, as she starts to "undress" or gets loose and opens up. He notices she's dangling her shoe off her foot. He understands that women, who dangle their shoes, while exposing the whole foot, can be an indicator of sexual curiosity. He remembered reading one of B Rich Scott's books, *"Foot Fetish: The Chronicles of a Gemini*", and recognized this sign of potential sexual interest.

He continued to stare as she spoke about her profession and other generic conversation. He could sense her getting hot, as she fans her face. She had on a black and white designer blouse that she needed to unbutton. She was getting hotter. This was the time for the guy, who she did not know, to use the metaphysical aspect of alcohol to bring her to a state of arousal. He realized by her shirt being unbuttoned and having her shoe hanging halfway off her foot that all these subtle, but important signs, were cues of undressing. And usually undressing in front of strangers creates a more enhanced level of attraction for both parties. All he would have to do now is say the right words to her to increase the level of apparent arousal.

The guy who she did not know, was well educated in the science of food and wanted to test out a different theory on elevating her sexual arousal level. He figured because they really did not know one another, a direct method would be too clumsy and unsexy, so he decided to experiment through food to see what kind of response he can get from this attractive woman. I told you this would not be a traditional health and fitness book.

The Role Food Plays in a Relationship (Dopamine)

What is Dopamine?

"Dopamine (DA, a contraction of 3,4-dihydroxyphenethylamine) is an organic chemical of the catecholamine and phenethylamine families. It functions both as a hormone and a neurotransmitter, and plays several important roles in the brain and body." - Wikipedia "Dopamine, serotonin, oxytocin, and endorphins are the quartet responsible for our happiness. Many events can trigger these neurotransmitters, but rather than being in the passenger seat, there are ways we can intentionally cause them to flow." -Oct 20, 2014, Huffington Post. Dopamine is a chemical reaction that can be created not only by food but by exercise and various legal and illegal drugs, e.g., dope.

In fact, some runners experience this thing called a "runner's high". I read an article in Scientific American by Judy Lavelle, Chemical & Engineering News that goes on to say: "After a nice long bout of aerobic exercise, some people experience what's known as a "runner's high": a feeling of euphoria coupled with reduced anxiety and a lessened ability to feel pain. For decades, scientists have associated this phenomenon with an increased level in the blood of βendorphins, opioid peptides thought to elevate the mood. Now, German researchers have shown the brain's endocannabinoid system—the same one affected by marijuana's Δ9-tetrahydrocannabinol (THC)—may also play a role in producing runner's high, at least in mice. (Proc. Natl. Acad. Sci. USA 2015, DOI: 10.1072/pnas.1514996112).

The researchers hit upon the endocannabinoid system as possibly being involved because they observed that endorphins can't pass through the blood-brain barrier, says team member Johannes Fuss, who's now at University Medical Center Hamburg-Eppendorf. On the other hand, a lipidsoluble endocannabinoid called anandamide—also found at high levels in people's blood after running—can travel from the blood into the brain, where it can trigger a natural high. "Yet no one had investigated the effects of endocannabinoids on behavior after running," Fuss says." Sidebar: CBD Oil is something that has hit the scene heavy and before you think that this may just be a fad it may be wise to do some research and see the benefits that this can have on not only your body but your spirit.

So now that I am done with the technical definition and terms of the word (for now) let me take you somewhere else real quick with it. Where do you think the word 'Dope' comes from? We can clearly see how the body and brain react to physical stimulation in a euphoric effect and I haven't even brought up what psychological things take place during sexual activities and sex, itself. As the cliché goes: we are what we eat. And that couldn't be truer in this case.

70% of our immune system is located within our gut, while 70% of our nervous system, which houses our neurotransmitters, not only in the brain but in the gut as well. That means dopamine, our favorite ‘mood enhancer’, is transported back and forth between the brain and the gut, and is heavily influenced by the nutrients that live in our guts. That's why probiotics are important. A lack of nutrition inevitably means a lack of dopamine, which translates best as a lack of happiness. That direct link from diet to happiness is enough of a reason for us to take a deeper look at the kind of food we are feeding our bodies, and whether we are unknowingly contributing to our lack of happiness by the neglect of our very own body.

Essentially, through the act of care for your own body, spirit, and health, you are able to control the desires of another person in order to attract and obtain your own core desires. Mind control at its finest. We have also heard the term "sugar rush" which is an experience of elevated energy after consuming a significant amount of sugar in a short period of time, often associated with hyperactive children and adults. There is usually a "crash" or feeling of extreme fatigue afterward. We know how powerful these chemical reactions are in the body and what it can cause a person to say or do. Some nutrition experts will have you believe that sugar is bad for you. There is no such thing as bad food. However, there are bad chemicals that we eat, which we call "food", and it is doing a doozy on society.

Remember earlier when I spoke about the time in my life when I loved Ramen noodles but began to question what this oily substance was? Well around the early 80's they were telling us butter was a bad thing and they introduced partially hydrogenated oil as a healthier option to reduce fat and help to lower cholesterol levels.

Sidebar: Men are not told how important cholesterol is in order to produce testosterone. Research that Bro! But what they failed to let the public know is that this was just a cheaper way to preserve products for a longer period of time, in exchange, this is causing a slew of health issues that have only increased over the years. Let's see what this oily substance really was and how "they" were able to classify this as a food.

Hydrogenation, complete or partial, is a chemical process in which hydrogen is added to liquid oils to turn them into a solid form. Partially hydrogenated fat molecules have trans fats, and they may be the worst type of fat you can consume. Let's see what the Mayo Clinic had to say about this.

What is Trans Fat?

"Some meat and dairy products contain small amounts of naturally occurring trans fat. But most trans fat is formed through an industrial process that adds hydrogen to vegetable oil, which causes the oil to become solid at room temperature. This partially hydrogenated oil is less likely to spoil, so foods made with it have a longer shelf life. Some restaurants use partially hydrogenated vegetable oil in their deep fryers because it doesn't have to be changed as often as other oils. The manufactured form of trans fat, known as partially hydrogenated oil, is found in a variety of food products, including: Baked goods. Most cakes, cookies, pie crusts and crackers contain shortening, which is usually made from partially hydrogenated vegetable oil.

Ready-made frosting is another source of trans fat. Snacks. Potato, corn and tortilla chips often contain trans fat. And while popcorn can be a healthy snack, many types of packaged or microwave popcorn uses Trans fat to help cook or flavor the popcorn. Fried food. Foods that require deep frying — French fries, doughnuts, and fried chicken — can contain trans fat from the oil used in the cooking process. Refrigerator dough. Products such as canned biscuits and cinnamon rolls often contain trans fat, as do frozen pizza crusts. Cream and margarine. Non Dairy coffee creamer and stick margarine also may contain partially hydrogenated vegetable oils.

Trans fat is considered by many doctors to be the worst type of fat you can eat. Unlike other dietary fats, trans fat — also called trans-fatty acids — both raise your LDL ("bad") cholesterol and lower your HDL ("good") cholesterol." What are the potential hormonal side effects that can take place when you introduce chemically created "foods" to your body? Way back in the day, we were told that your DNA cannot be changed, but modern science has now proven that to be untrue and are changing people's DNA on a regular basis.

Sidebar: Did you know that fasting for 72 hours can help regenerate your entire DNA system for the better? Not only does food change your DNA but the bodily fluids that people in sexual relationships exchange with one another can also change the DNA of a person as well. This is why some couples who have been in a relationship for a long time start to look like one another. This is where we will get into the sexual relationship side of metaphysics, now that we know and can agree metaphysics is a real thing.

Sexual Transmutation

What happens when a man impregnates a woman? You are probably like, "Dude, I picked up this book to get my damn body in shape, what the hell is all this?" Trust me; you are in the right place… I got you, but let me continue. When a man impregnates a woman, not only is that sperm powerful enough to create life but in many cases, it is powerful enough to make a child that looks like HIM out of that woman's own body. The more powerful the man's sperm is the more physical characteristics that the child will have.

Think about that for a second. So if the sperm is powerful enough to create a person that looks like you from another whole person that does not look like you, what do you think it is doing to the woman's DNA? In my series UnF**k Your Life, in the book UnF**k Your Feelings, I will go deeper into the sexual metaphysical side of this, but for now, I will just touch the surface here.

So in fact, nature has ALWAYS been able to manipulate DNA but we were told otherwise. What else has been hidden from us? I can go into how the energy of a man through sex is passed on through to the woman, and in turn, she starts becoming more and more like that male. One example is when she is in an argument with you she is channeling through her, the masculine energy of her past lovers, including your own energy. She is literally becoming you and if you do not know how to handle that, this may change the dynamic of a relationship. In fact, at some point it ALWAYS changes the dynamic of a relationship, but that's to be expected. The man's job is to reign that spirit back in. I urge men to put down the soy!!!!

"Clean Foods"

There are so many people out there that think that they are eating "clean", because they are eating all the foods that are low in fat and are low in cholesterol. They are eating all of their vegetables and are staying away from dairy. They cut the sugar and salt out, but fail to understand terms like sucrose and monosodium glutamate. A person who does not understand chemicals or how to properly read a nutrition label is helpless from the deception and schemes from these food companies to keep you addicted to the "product". In my opinion, it is better to go with the actual salt, the actual sugar and the full-fat option (in most cases), instead of the cheaper chemicals they use to substitute and trick your taste buds.

Some of these chemicals used to substitute sugar have not only been proven to cause cancer but have also been proven to increase the chances of diabetes, which is usually the reason why people go with these substitute options in the first place, to avoid that. Here is a US News article published in April of 2018 about this very same problem. "As diabetes and obesity become a rising worldwide health concern there has been an increased awareness of environmental factors, such as diet, that are contributing to the problem," the study says.

"However, it was not until recently that the negative impact of consuming non-caloric artificial sweeteners in place of sugar had been increasingly recognized as a potential contributor to the dramatic increase in diabetes and obesity, along with the associated complications." The results of the study suggest artificial sweeteners alter how bodies process fat and obtain energy. Additionally, researchers discovered acesulfame potassium appeared to accumulate in the blood, with increased amounts having more harmful effects on cells that line blood vessels.

One of the authors, Brian Hoffmann, assistant professor in the department of biomedical engineering at the Medical College of Wisconsin and Marquette University, said sugar replacements aren't a solution to the diabetes and obesity epidemic. "Despite the addition of these non-caloric artificial sweeteners to our everyday diets, there has still been a drastic rise in obesity and diabetes," Hoffmann said in the release.

"In our studies, both sugar and artificial sweeteners seem to exhibit negative effects linked to obesity and diabetes, albeit through very different mechanisms from each other."

It saddens me to see people thinking they are doing the right thing in order to be a better version of themselves, but they have to basically be a scientist, biochemist and damn near a detective in order to halfway be able to do any of this right. Even when people trust someone like a nutritionist, who is supposed to be an expert in the field of food and nutrition. They advise people on what to eat in order to lead a healthy lifestyle or achieve a specific health-related goal. The problem is that most of these "experts" don't even know what the hell they are doing.

Sidebar: Have you noticed how many people in the medical industry (which is supposed to be concerned with your health) smoke cigarettes, especially nurses and doctors? That's just wild as fuck to me.

But I digress. Too many times we just focus solely on a person's weight and not actually what they look like on the inside. Not a lot of people understand how important their blood labs are in the equation, and that can be problematic. If you do not know the right questions to ask then you may not know where or how to tackle the root problem. As a person who is extremely passionate about health, I have tried to teach and have always urged my clients to learn how to read lab work when they get their blood drawn. It is also important to know what labs to ask for. Many doctors will not check for even the most fundamental hormonerelated things to your overall health and well-being unless you tell them to do it, or unless something is wrong and they cannot find a cookie-cutter solution to the problem.

Testosterone and estrogen levels should always be checked for men starting around the age of 30, so that you have a baseline to compare from. From that point, hormone levels should be checked yearly, in some cases, every six months. Many hormone therapists and urologists understand this, but if you aren't recommended from your primary care doctor to one of these specialists, you may not know that you even need this kind of physician. The professionals that you trust to have your best interest in regard to health, unfortunately, have another agenda for you. Again, without going too much down that path, I will just say, if you can at least understand the outline that I am about to give to you on how to change your lifestyle, you will have yet, another tool to significantly keep yourself from depending on the people that do not care if you are actually well.

If your food labels have ingredients that you have to Google in order to recognize what they are, then that may be a product you may want to think twice about consuming. Let me be clear, there are plenty of ingredients that you may actually not understand or cannot even pronounce, but they are good for you. Most vitamins in its original compound language are listed and they may look foreign to a person who does not understand that. Example, Vitamin D is commonly known as ergocalciferol (Vitamin D2) and cholecalciferol (Vitamin D3). For those starting on their fitness journeys or even those that have been on this journey for a while, but have been stuck spinning their wheels, I would suggest this simple tip that will take some discipline. If your nutrition label has more than five ingredients, do not consume it. You may not be ready in your discipline, or may not be knowledgeable enough to have discernment when it comes to what may be preventing you from excelling in your fitness journey. I said this before and will stress this again. THERE ARE NO BAD FOODS! But most foods are now chemicals.

Most fruit flavors are not made with real fruit, they are simply created with food coloring and chemicals. If you are going to consume a product that has a “sugar-free” label, there is going to be a trade-off that may not be worth it. I would instruct my clients to take the product that actually has real sugar instead of those poisonous artificial sweeteners. I would always go with the labels that say salt rather than a product that says salt substitute.

Why? Because sometimes a saltsubstitute has actually more sodium per serving than actual salt. That's a trick that they hope many consumers do not catch...And they don't! Sidebar: A lot of people think that salt and sodium are the same. They are not. That's like saying sugar and sweeteners are the same. Two totally different things. When many people buy a food product and look for salt, they look in the ingredients. That's where most people stop and will not do any further research. They should have paid more attention to the sodium number, that's more of the issue, because a product can contain salt and have 10 mg of sodium per serving. Another product may not have the word "salt" listed but have 1000 mg per serving of sodium. Can you see how dangerous and dishonest that is? There is a reason why companies can get away with this. When you understand what a lobbyist is, the reasons will make more sense. You are going to have to do that research on your own though.

Sidebar: Don't worry, I didn't forget about the couple I started to discuss earlier. I am letting him do his thing so we have some content to break down. We will circle back and check in on those two later.

Energetic Class

When you are around people that are doing the same thing as you, it's sometimes hard to see how you may fall into a rhythm of consistency and not out of free will (although technically it is free will). You all start to like the same things, talk the same way, and eat the same things. There is a reason why conventional wisdom says, "Birds of a feather tend to flock together". Take a look at the five closest people to you in your life currently and there are probably a lot of similarities when it comes to social class, educational class and financial class.

Something people rarely think about though is the spiritual (or energetic) class that they also associate themselves with and how this affects one's well-being. This can be another puzzle you need to learn how to put together when it comes to your overall wellness. When we sit down to eat with our close friends, there is a social bonding that takes place unconsciously. Everyone is sharing the same frequency of energy; this relates to the comradely part of the experience. In groups where the energy is in cohesion and the attitudes are in alignment, that food that you are eating now subconsciously becomes part of the "tribal culture".

For many people that sit down and break bread together, it feels like a family experience. To many, it can take them to a time that's nostalgic. Even if you have never experienced a traditional family dinner before, when a group of people sit down to eat delicious food, it causes reactions to take place in the neurological sensors and the bodies' chemistry. Here come those endorphins and dopamines again. So, because this experience feels so good, it is easy to over-eat foods that may not be the best of options. And because everyone else is doing it, this may have you participating in these experiences more often, because the group's energy is so great to be part of.

If you do not think the energy in a group of people eating together is a real thing, let me paint you a picture. I will pinpoint where the energy shifts and tell you why consciously and subconsciously it makes some people feel uncomfortable. Let this be clear because it will help you throughout your fitness journey, *sometimes you have to break what is most comfortable for you to have success*.

When a group of peers sits down to break bread together, there is a giving and a mutual understanding that we are all here to have a good time and to share an experience together. Food just happens to be the commonality in which we all decided to partake in. Now it does not matter if it is two or twenty people. When everyone is acting in accordance with the same vibe, one person can disrupt that group's flow by not eating. That one lack of action (no eating) seems to be taking AWAY from the group's normal exchange of energy.

And in fact, metaphysically speaking, it actually does!

I rarely go out to eat because of how anal and specific I am when it comes to food. So when I do go out with friends to eat, those who know me and know how I rock, they love watching me order, because it's straight theatre! There was a time where I used to be the biggest fast food and restaurant junkie. I was extra with it. I do not do normal "average-people" things; I go big and extreme with things. I had a huge appetite for both life and food. In terms of food, I would do things like, go to IHOP and order breakfast, lunch AND dinner in one sitting. Then an hour later take down a whole large pizza. There was one year where I lived on nothing but Chinese food for that whole year…Literally. There were no other foods brought into the equation during that year. There were times in my life that I would drink bottles and bottles of two-liter sodas daily.

I had a diet that consisted of pizza, French fries, ice cream, more pizza, pasta, subs, cool ranch Doritos, snickers, butterfingers, the orange-flavored Hostess cupcakes, you name it…I was on it. But check this out…I WAS NEVER FAT! I may have had more body fat on my frame than I wanted to have, but I was never, at any time, at risk of being even remotely obese. I definitely have to thank my genetics on some level for my body type. However, I also feel that if I were to eat the same things I was eating in the late 90's -early 2000's, I would have a whole host of health issues today, because the food is not of the same quality and standard of production that it was back then.

I started changing my diet right around the time the foods were starting to be created in labs and probably around the same time ya moms created you, lol. So people who DO NOT really knows me, do not understand that if I do go out to eat, it's going to get weird for everyone involved... Real fast!

I have been out to birthday dinners in restaurants and when I started to order people at the table, which I did not know me, would look at me like "WTF?"

I have to know how the food was prepared because I do not use microwaves. It must be cooked on the grill, oven or stovetop.

I have to know if the meat was pre-seasoned. I know that most restaurants marinate their chicken to save time and to seal in the flavor, but most places do this with a bunch of sodium-laced seasonings. So unless they use a clean undressed bird, in which you can season at the time of order, I stay away from ordering chicken from any place.

Steaks are safer for me because most are usually clean, but not always, so I still have to ask. Even with that being said, I have to make sure that they prepare it clean, meaning, no salt, no pepper, no butter, no seasoning of any kind while being cooked. If the place does not serve steak then I most likely will watch everyone else eat. Because of the energy and the synchronicity that is taking place with the chewing and the taste buds being titillated, there is an intangible thing that happens when people eat together that you just can't put your finger on, but its there.

When you are not contributing, and are not sharing in that experience, you are taking away from the energy of that experience and not adding to it. Subconsciously, people feel it, but again, it's intangible so they may not know why they feel the way they do. Internally, this can create a feeling of people not liking you.

Let's go deeper.

A person who does not give too much care about their health, more often than not, will tend to associate with others who do not care too much about their health either. With that being said, it's not too farfetched to say, people who are not mindful on how they eat, will often not care about how their body looks.

Let me rephrase this.

They *may* care, but aren't prepared to do anything tangible about it, like get a trainer, eat healthier, exercise. Instead, they will always have an *EXCUSE* why they cannot succeed or are slacking in their fitness journey, "It's too hard." "It costs too much." "My body is in pain."Blah. Blah. Blah.... Cry me a fucking river why don't ya.

Conversely, when a person who *DOES* cares about their body/health, enters into a setting in which no one is really being held accountable on how they eat or what the fuck they look like, it can subconsciously make some people uncomfortable. And this can *consciously* put some people into a mindset of, "*Who does he/she think they are? They think they're better than me?*" If you are that person who refuses to eat poor choices of food when the group is eating, you unknowingly can be looked at as a "downer" because it can be perceived as you not being part of "OUR tribe."

Some people may actually think that you (healthy/fit person) are trying to shame them just for being present and they will feel insulted. Do you know how many times I have entered a building and people have told me, "Bro, you're making us look bad." I smile, but in my mind I say, "Well, do something about it!" (I do actually say this to people now, jokingly of course, then hand them my business card) Only 1% follows through, because most people do not want to do the work, refer back to previous excuses.

I tell my female clients who have been overweight for a long period of time to pay attention to how your friends start to act as you go deeper into your fitness journey and the results start becoming visible. Remember, birds of feather usually flock together, so there is a likely chance that these friends are overweight as well. Sometimes these friends will seemingly be proud of your integrity and accomplishments. Don't be fooled! Some of them harbor hearts filled with jealousy. You can tell by the fakeness on how they compliment you. *"Hey girl, don't lose too much weight"* Bye HATER! This is something you must be aware of once you start becoming strong in your discipline.

A person without this level of discipline or one that tries to undermine your progress will say something like, "Hey, why can't you just go with the flow and take one day off? It's not going to affect you. You are too concerned about your health; we all got to go sometime. You might as well experience life's pleasures." What they are really saying is, "Hey, you're making me look bad and I do not want to be held accountable for the bad nutrition decisions I have made in my life right now." You are basically throwing all their poor decisions in their face.

Personally, I am aware of the effects my way of eating may have on others. I have witnessed this many times. I have been known to bring food from home to restaurants so that I can keep up and enjoy participating with the group. I have attended other people's cookouts with my own meat that I cooked when I got there. I get strange looks, oh fucking well! There was a sub shop that I used to go to all the time before I stopped eating out. They had a charcoal grill they used to make their barbeque chicken on. One day, I took my marinated chicken from home to the sub shop and had them place my chicken on their industrial-sized charcoal grill. I had them make it into a sub using their sub roll, tomatoes and onion. I did this kind of thing often.

I have plenty of interesting food stories but I will share this last one. I loved buying uncooked pizza from Whole Foods that would need to be cooked in the oven at home. I would preheat the oven to 375° for about 10 minutes, undo the packaging and place that beauty in the oven. My house would smell like a pizzeria. I was in New Orleans at this particular time and did not have access to an oven at the place where I was staying, but I wanted my pizza cooked immediately. There happened to be a Domino's pizza shop not too far from me. I walked in, I told the guy behind the counter that I would give him $5 if he ran my pizza through their oven. The dude looked at me kind of strange, but was like, "Fuck it!" Domino's ovens are unique. They are equipped with the rolling racks, which to me, seems to add more of a crisper crust. The pizza that day was exceptionally good. To many, this may sound "extra," extreme or like "I'm doing too much."

I have been doing this for over 20 years, I am strong in my discipline and comfortable enough to express to people the way I choose to eat whether they get it or not.

I make no apologies for it.

This is how I go about my lifestyle and it makes it easier for people to respect once they see where your line is drawn in the sand. Make the decision now where you want that line to be drawn and stick to it. Again, none of this will be easy. If it was, everyone would be doing it.

I can only promise you that it will be worth it. In my personal opinion, getting the nutrition part down is the hardest part and takes the most discipline. Some people have a problem with the actual working out part, but even if you are a person that takes your workouts to the extreme, the max you will do in the gym will never equate to the amount of extreme discipline it takes not to fuck up your diet.

Let's say you are training in the gym for 2 hours (which is way too long for the average person) two hours is nothing compared to the other 22 hours in which you need to make sure you are eating what you are supposed to and making sure you are not doing anything to set you back. Now back to how food plays a part in your spirit. Although I do not believe in bad foods, I do believe some foods have higher and lower vibrations than others. What that basically means is that there are some foods that are going to not only feed your body, but feed your soul as well. And depending on that food's vibration, you may be feeding your soul some bullshit!

Just like all bodies are not created the same, the same can be said for food. All foods are not created the same. Some foods are prepared with more love than others. Some people serve you food from a bitter or depressed spirit. The transfer of energy from one living organism to another is quite fascinating when you see it manifest in real time.

Imagine a person is preparing food for a funeral, and the person who is preparing the food has a heavy heart because of their loss. It's fair to say that everyone who eats this food at the repass will already be mourning to some extent but will not notice such a huge shift in their emotional status. Now let's just say this same food is left over and is given to someone who has no attachment to the person who has passed away. This person is in good spirits, but after eating this food, a day or two later, there is a minor shift in this person's spirit. Nothing too disruptive, and to the untrained spirit, it may seem like nothing at all. But this is a thing. And it is real.

Toxic foods still have to be broken down and it takes a lot of energy for your body to break certain toxins down, which weakens your body from being able to fuel and nourish other parts that are important like the mind which controls every aspect of the body. I would jump out on a limb and say that a majority of mental diseases may be circumvented through diet. But I am not at liberty to say that, so I digress. This will be the perfect time to check back in on that couple and see how they are making out. The last thing we should remember was that the guy understood the dynamics and the metaphysics behind food and the chemicals disguised as food. He was going to put some of what he knew into action in regard to this pretty woman that he wanted to get to know and eventually sleep with.

Let's pick it back up from where we left off... He knows that there is a better chance of taking her home if he can get her to change the location of where she is now. Even if it's just a small change in scenery. Any cooperation from her would be an advantage for him. He asks the attractive lady if she is hungry and if she would like to eat. He is hoping she cannot resist the offer, because if she accepts, the seduction can continue, but also a new game will soon begin. She tilts her head to the side while brushing her hair out of her face and says, "Yes!" "I know this nice restaurant not too far from here. I can have you back before your friends even miss you." He said. She looks back at her friends on the dance floor and they are surrounded by some other guys flirting, laughing and lying, she figures. She says, "No worries, they are busy, I will text them and let them know I'm headed out." He grabs her hand and they go.

Sidebar: There are certain foods that are known as aphrodisiacs. An aphrodisiac is an agent (such as a food or drug) that arouses or is held to arouse sexual desire. He knows the power of food. There was a time back in the day, where men would use a product called Cantharidin a.k.a., Spanish Fly to make women horny. It has been used for thousands of years as a sexual stimulant. I want to stress, this was way different than the date rape drug (Rohypnol or "roofies"), no one would pass out or do anything they were not aware of doing, but this product was poisonous in large doses and still usually done without consent or the woman being aware.

He orders her steak and oysters, along with a glass of red wine and dark chocolate dipped strawberries. He feeds her a strawberry as they both take sips of wine. He starts complimenting her and stares intensely at her mouth. She tells him a little bit of what she does for work and about her interests, but this is just social politics at this point, however, he appears locked in on every word that escapes from her delectable lips. She is also engaged and is enjoying the conversation's flow and the energy that he is stirring beneath the surface. She doesn't know why she feels so comfortable, but the more he speaks, the more she wants to submerge in his words. He makes a comment about the ancient history of red Ginseng and the mysterious properties that this herb is supposed to contain. This piqued her curiosity. "Tell me more" she anxiously replies.

He explained into detail which made her want to try this mysterious elixir. By chance, he just happened to have some Ginseng with him. He reached into his pocket and pulled out a small glass vial that was sealed with a green cap at the top. The liquid was a cola color and the label had Chinese writing on it. He asked her if she wanted to find out what it tasted like. With eyes wide open, she licked her lips. "Absolutely!" was her reply.

He placed the bottle in her pretty manicured hands and she took a sip. Her face scrunched up as the bitter liquid hit her tongue. She was taken aback by the taste. She was not prepared to be hit with that kind of power. You have to prepare for the taste of Ginseng, it's an acquired taste. The bitterness was followed by a sweet taste of honey in an effort to cut down the bite from the powerful root. He noticed her initial expression, but she was a trooper about hers and continued to down the rest of the tiny bottle that seemed to go on forever. She licked her lips and the shoe that was dangling off her foot dropped to the floor.

What a lovely sound he thought. At that moment the entree had arrived at the table and they partook in the meal. Not many words were being spoken, but there was DEFINITELY communication going on back and forth. He watched as she placed the meat on her fork and then into her mouth. He thought about what it would feel like for his meat to slide in between her cheeks. He knew it was only a matter of time before his vision became reality. (Metaphysics}He meditated and envisioned this exact scenario days earlier through a ritual of *Sex Magic.*

Sex Magic is a ritualistic practice within a spiritual pursuit for the purpose of manifesting the desired result through visualization during the act of sex or a sexual act. He understood the science and the Universal Laws behind such projections and manifestations. He also understood the power and energy that his body would absorb by retaining his seed and not ejaculating. He understood that every time a man releases his seed (semen), life force escapes from his spirit. He had already seen her in his bedroom, through meditation, with the lit candles dancing in the background on the walls, as her sexy ass silhouette bounced up and down on his hard dick. His penis would soon penetrate her vaginal area but she would have no idea how deep his erection would penetrate her spirit.

Sidebar: Metaphysically speaking, it has been argued that a teaspoon of semen is equal to a pint of blood, as far as how the body and spirit feel energetically. There is a minimum time frame in order to gain maximum potential with seed retention, but most men cannot go a day without ejaculation.

As they get comfortable, she begins to lustfully doze in and out of a drunken trance, carefully removing one shoe after the other. The endless flow of red wine and Raspberry-Vanilla Martini on her breath, along with goose bumps across her bare silky smooth thighs, says all but "I'm ready to be fucked." As she moves, he is carefully observing her imminent acquiesce to his every whim. Her plan is working. This was the moment she had been carefully plotting since she saw him walking into the bar earlier that evening. Just as bad as he wanted and planned to get her from the moment their eyes locked, she too, had been yearning, and plotting, to seduce him into a hypnotic trance and have her way with him.

Fluent in the language of energy and social cues, he slyly makes note of her vibe as he reaches over her lap to his Gin & Cranberry tonic sitting on the armrest. He offers her another drink, to which she accepts. Hot, steamy passion is now full steam ahead, as she eloquently, yet assertively pulls him deeper and deeper into a trance. In such a dull grey, watered-down world, she is the spice of life and new energy.

A Goddess in a Christian church, a witch in a world of robots. She is an ethereal Wonder Woman who knows how to get what she wants. And what she wants right now is right in front of her waiting on him to make a move. With tools like Tantric, Kama Sutra and Sex Magic in her "seduction" arsenal, there's no man that could stand a chance against her sexualprowess.

Sex Magic can be used with another or against another, together as a couple, or separately as an individual, and is an act of intention and attention.

It was fully her intention to get him within her zone, right where she wants him and through Sex Magic this would be the perfect time. As a self-proclaimed sex nerd, she knows the subtle art of careful seduction in such a way that doesn't interrupt the traditional "game" of masculine nature and the need to initiate the pursuit of prey. She knows all too well the idea of becoming the "prey" in order to catch her own prey, and how to strategically place herself in a position to which she attracts anything and more importantly, anyone, her heart desires.

She knows this all too well firsthand how effective diet is when it comes to not only herself but also her sexual partners and the spiritual connection shared between them.

From promoting the increase of dopamine through sensual experiences, to controlling the function of the amygdala that processes these and other internal emotions, her plan would soon be realized as he stands in front of her, ready to devour and spoil her in ways only a master seductress would expect.

The Spirit Tantric practice is an Eastern sexual modality that promotes the clearing and healing of clogged energy in the form of repressed sexual trauma. It is used as a holistic health tool, as well as a powerful, intimate boosting and meditative aphrodisiac. Kama Sutra is an ancient Indian Sanskrit text on sexuality, eroticism and emotional fulfillment in life. The text-based practice is written as a guide to the "art-of-living" well, the nature of love, finding a life partner, maintaining one's love life, and other aspects pertaining to pleasure-oriented faculties of human life.

Kama Sutra is the oldest surviving Hindu text on erotic love. And those who study and implement its wisdom are sure to find the soulfulfilling, new heights they are seeking within the realm of pleasure. In terms of pleasure, the 3rd eye, or “pineal gland” is what houses your neurotransmitters, and your amygdala, which controls your dopamine levels every time you engage in a pleasurable activity. Pleasurable activities such as sex, eating, shopping, etc., are all closely related and controlled by the amygdala within your pineal gland.

With food, your pineal gland remains either calcified or decalcified, depending on the type of diet you consume. Whole, nutritious foods and other nutrients that I cannot reveal here can help decalcify your pineal gland which clears toxic debris from the region of your brain that controls your spiritual insight and evolution. That means there is a direct link from diet to your spirit that is undeniable and affects not only your internal self but also your external self, including lifestyle factors such as diet, fitness and overall health. It can have you choosing who you decide to keep in your life or not.

If you pay attention, you can make a direct correlation from the quality and type of foods some neighborhoods have to the social mentality these neighborhoods also share. But more importantly, you will feel the energy that is shared throughout the neighborhood. Understand that people smarter than you DO have a plan. Please do not be shocked here. Foods are pushed into certain neighborhoods to keep the spirit of that community fucked up and destitute.

Food is life, and I mean this spiritually, mentally, physically, emotionally, logically and LITERALLY!

A romantic relationship can be destroyed by the wrong food (chemicals). Look at my last sentence and repeat this like a Goddamn mantra because that should be your mantra. "Food is life, and I mean this spiritually, mentally, physically, emotionally, logically and LITERALLY!"

Food directly affects stress levels as well as your coping capacity for normal daily stresses of life from work, family and other factors. Diet can affect everything from your health and emotional state, to your sexual fulfillment. But being well versed in Tantra, Sex Magic and other modalities sometimes isn't even enough to penetrate through the toxicity that develops from the environment in which we mostly have full control of. From the way we eat to the water we drink, to the lifestyle vices we take on like smoking, drinking etc., they all contribute to our overall well-being in life.

When we eat right, we live right. When we eat well, we feel well. It's that simple.

The Physical

When we talk about fitness and nutrition we have to understand that the body is an amazing, complicated, co-dependent machine that is created for optimum performance, and optimum performance is determined by how all parts are working independently, as well as cohesively. Full range of motion in all body parts, including veins, muscles and bones are vital for the body to be able to do everything it's physically capable of doing. Sometimes when we stop working on certain parts of the body, it weakens other body parts.

This can cause stronger body parts to pull more load than they are supposed to pull in order to compensate. In order to create better spirits we need to build better bodies. This is where working out and physical activity plays a big part. Anyone that has a personal training certification or has done any studying of the human body can attest to how intricate the body's' design is. There are many ways to get the body and the spirit in sync with one another. Exercise and sex are two of the simplest ways to align the two. I have already spoken in great detail about sex, so let's take a look at the actual training of the body.

Personally, the working out part of staying fit and healthy is the easiest part for me. There are plenty that will disagree and I feel them, but the hardest part about working out to me, is wanting to get into my car and make that drive to the gym. But as soon as I am actually in the gym, it's time! Some people are self-conscious about going into the gym because they are insecure about their bodies and do not want anyone else to see them or to judge them. This can be crippling and debilitating and can create psychological blocks that can keep someone from even starting their journey.

One piece of advice that I can suggest is to do some light training in the privacy of your own home or a friend's home. You do not need expensive machines or even a gym membership, to be honest. I am going to give you a list of some simple things you can have in your arsenal to help you begin your journey. Most people love a mat to put on the ground instead of having to be on the floor or the ground. (I personally do not care, I will train in the dirt if need be) some sneakers to train in, some shorts and a comfortable t-shirt, a jump rope, a 5 lb dumbbell and some water. I can get you in great physical condition with just those materials. A lot of the populations are not trying to be bodybuilders, many just want to be able to fit into their clothes and have a little bit of muscle tone when they go to the beach.

Exercises like jumping jacks, blurpees, mountain climbers and push-ups are great for conditioning in helping the body to drop actual fat off your frame. Running drills are extremely helpful as well. I like to have my clients do 100-yard dashes to get the most from a running drill. My drills are quite intense, but the workouts are so powerful, that days later your body is still in the state of arousal and calories are still being burned at an efficiently higher rate. There are hundreds of thousands of people that do not go to a commercial gym and look better than those that do. So, if not having access to a gym is not the real issue, then what is?

NO PAIN, NO GAIN (I'm talking about Discipline)

That expression, "No pain, no gain" was coined probably by someone who didn't understand what that fully means. It sounds all good and everything in the "Bro" world, but many people who workout do not subscribe to or even know what the Bro world is when it comes to training. I will just say this, although a lot of things in this world can be proven to get you results, there are better, more efficient, and SAFER ways to maximize your results.

If you think the more pain you inflict on your body, the more gains you are going to receive, you may want to think again! You can actually be causing more damage to your body. There is a minor exception to that statement, though, and that applies if you are using performance-enhancing drugs. I will not get into that here. That's a whole book on its own, but I digress.

Although it is true that in order for your muscles to grow, they actually DO have to be damaged. Muscles grow when that muscle is torn and has taken time to repair and recover. This is how new and bigger muscles are formed. The problem is, many people over train and do not give their body enough time to recover and in turn, they create pain in their bodies and think that's a good thing because they "feel the burn." Feeling the burn is not always a good thing. And here is something that you should always remember when it comes to training. The nervous system is extremely vital in causing new muscle growth.

If you do not allow your nervous system to rest or are consistently overtraining, you can actually halt your progress and start to regress. Let me say that again...Sounds crazy as fuck!

True story Bro, but no, if you are training too much and not allowing your body to get the proper rest and nutrition, the gains that you actually did obtain, can diminish, quickly!

This is what I mean when I say that a lot of people think they are doing the right thing. They keep spinning their wheels but not really getting anywhere. Why is this so damn complicated, right? Well, I wish I could tell you that it wasn't, but if you have made it this far in the book, you can see that it is a process. It may not be easy, hopefully, with this information, I have provided you with, and it will help with your transition.

My intent was for you to have a different perspective on health and fitness and if you tell me that you don't, you're lying to yourself (not me, YOU!) I want to stress that the most important key to all of this is discipline. Discipline is what it will take for you to begin and continue on this journey and make it a lifestyle. There is a lot of trauma that prevents some of us from being the greatest versions of ourselves and there are layers to this. How do we know what trauma is fucking us up if we have no idea what trauma we have buried deep down inside of us?

The Devil We Don't Know

Living your life at its highest climax doesn't just start with lifestyle adjustments like eating and working out, although by doing so, you are helping the bottom line. Truth is, health & wellness is a deeply rooted tree. The root of that tree begins not outside of you, but INSIDE of you. The internal workings of who you are, are what creates health & life, and similarly, creates death and trauma as well. Many people look good on the outside, but the truth is, being thin naturally leads people to believe that thin means healthy when in fact, that couldn't be further from the truth. If we wore our internal selves on the outside of our bodies, many of us would look like a zombie straight out of The Walking Dead.

Luckily though, we don't look like what we've been through, so it saves us a great deal of necessary beauty sleep. However, just because we do not essentially "look" like what we've been through, truth be told, our past trauma still affects our practical day-to-day lives in ways most of us do not understand even as full-grown adults. Imagine a 5-year-old child growing up neglected and abused by a single mother, who is unable to give the necessary love and affection needed for the developing confidence of that growing boy.

Now, that young boy must learn to seek comfort through outside sources as he grows and matures. That comfort may now come through sources such as sex, and yes, even food. In an attempt to comfort the neglected emotions he feels wallowing inside of himself, he turns to food as a way to not only fill that void but also to distract himself from the love he lacked as a child. That coping mechanism may eventually turn into an eating disorder such as binging or "emotional eating" which also eventually leads to obesity and not to mention, functioning depression. Or, maybe your past trauma wasn't THAT horrible.

Maybe you were a child in a loving home with attentive parents who made sure you were loved and supported with the necessary tools and regimes it takes to properly raise a child. Maybe in an effort to practice good parenting, with pure intentions, your mother often told you to "eat all your food" at dinner before leaving the table. Sound familiar? It made sense to you as a child, because your mother only wants the best for you, she only wants you to get the nutrients your body needs in order to develop properly. So who are you to argue?

Mom knows best, right? Well, it's always interesting to watch how a child processes info received during childhood. Now you grow up with the mentality that someone else knows your body and your limits better than you do, so even though your stomach says you are full and have had enough, you finish what's on your plate and ignore your own intuitive signals because…. "Mom knows best".

Trauma doesn't always have to be acute or dark. Sometimes, the subtle advice given against our very own intuit system leaves us with limiting beliefs that hinder our own greatness as we attempt to evolve into the masterpiece we were born to be. That childhood advice to "eat all the food on your plate" may have caused you to learn how to ignore your own intuition, and even on the practical side, it may have very well increased your stomach's capacity for food, eventually leading to weight gain and the vicious cycle of eating more food than your bodily functions require.

Point is, doing your shadow-work and exploring your internal self to uproot the limiting beliefs based on childhood trauma or simply unlearning "bad advice" (I'm sure Mama meant well), is extremely important in achieving even your most practical health and fitness goals. Once those unproductive roots are dug up, the "branch" work you do in the gym and in the kitchen will lead to bearing the fruit of that tree. But it starts within you, first and foremost.

As an Ordained Fitness Minister, I have trained many men and women in the art of giving up that which no longer serves you. It's extremely common to see people over-extending themselves for years until they come to a professional like myself, who is able to get to the root of the problem and create a plan that leads to not only internal healing but also gives practical results you can see in the mirror. Emotional eating does not start nor end on its own. Procrastination, especially as it relates to gym consistency, does not start nor end on its own. Even the diet you consume does not start nor end on its own.

You are conditioned to eat and love certain foods. Now you must re-condition yourself to do better, to eat better, and to live better. But, it's up to you. YOU must make that choice once and for all, and once you do that I can help you. Are you ready to make a change, from the inside out? What is stopping you? Think about it. I'm here for you when you are ready to make that move.

My job as an Ordained Fitness Minister is to figure out what is blocking you from being able to start your journey and helping you continue this journey until you feel strong enough to walk it on your own. I have helped many clients not only change their bodies but have helped them change their minds. I have designed warriors and consider myself King of the Beast Mode because you have to be able to tame the beast in order to maintain order. Like I said in the beginning, there is way too much information that I have in mind to express at one time. I wanted this to be a short easy read. I have covered a lot of topics here and will have a lot more to come in the future.

For immediate services or if you would like to be a part of my program in with I can help you through a 12-week programs that guides you through the training, meal prep, spiritual and emotional side to get you off the hamster wheel once and for all so that you FINALLY have the tools to free yourself you can visit my website www.brichscott.com

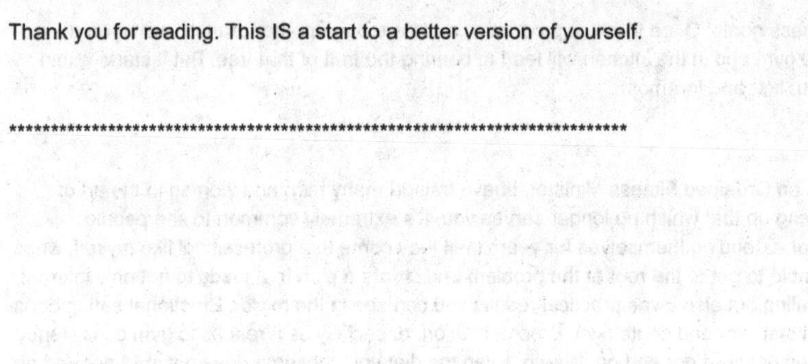

Thank you for reading. This IS a start to a better version of yourself.

****

Wait .... What? Something is missing you say? The conclusion of what?

Ooh, the story about the couple. No, I did not forget, they will be the subject of the next book in this series "UnF**k Your Feelings" A holistic and practical look at emotion. If you think this was an interesting and unconventional read, this was a child's book compared to what will be in that book. Here's an excerpt from the next book in the series "UnF**k Your Feelings" A holistic and practical look at emotion.

*Revised chapter

UnF**k Covid

Towards the tail end of 2019, many people experienced a certain level of sickness and fatigue that they have never felt before. Many people chopped it up to an extreme case of the flu, but there were a few people that knew something was seriously wrong. I was one of those people at the time that did not think too much of it. It was the night before Christmas Eve, I was on my way to the airport. I had an afternoon flight to catch on standby. I was headed to Atlanta to spend the holiday out there. A week prior I had been excited about the upcoming NBA Christmas Day line-up. That was going to be the best gift as far as I was concerned. I could not wait to wake up to a large cooked breakfast, presents and the first game at noon to start. I had it all planned out.

Before I got to the airport I was thinking to myself that, "If I do not get on this first flight, I may just have to tap out, because I barely felt good enough to take this one. If you know anything about flying standby, you may have to wait all day at the airport and still not get a seat. But I made a promise. Initially, I did not think too much of me not feeling well, I just thought that this was an extremely major cold. I do not feel that it reached "flu" status until I actually got to the airport. I felt like my body temperature had shot up.

I had concluded that perhaps the sudden increase of heat that I was experiencing had come from the cold wintery weather. By taking public transportation, I had exposed myself to Boston's Bully winter weather. Waiting on a train or bus in the winter in Boston is no joke!

Going through the TSA in itself can make a person sick. So imagine my frustration when one of the belts to run the baggage security checks were down. It was like watching a circus but none of these clowns were funny, at all! I just wanted to sit down at this point. After undressing three layers of clothes (exaggerating, but still) I managed to find the strength to make it to my gate just as the flight was boarding. I looked on the standby last at the gate to see if my name appeared anywhere on the list.

Not there. I went to approach the gate attendant but the line had already a few people in it, and just like up front at security, there was chaos back here as well. Christmas holiday, ya know? I dropped my luggage to keep my spot in line, and then took a seat. I watched all the families and individuals' faces. Some were happy, some were aggravated, and some were talking about what they wanted for Christmas. All these sounds were fading in and out; I could hear all conversations clearly, while some just sounded just like background noise. I heard this all at the same time.

I felt like I was out of it. I was exhausted and just wanted to sit there and rest. I watched the line for customer service dwindle down; I approached, with my lethargic body, to the gate. My sickness had escalated rather quickly. That was odd, but I still was not overly concerned. I asked the person at the counter if there was any way that I would be able to get a seat on this flight.

I was told that this flight was overbooked and some of the people who had a purchased seat may not even get on this flight. Say less I thought. I proceeded to take my ass right back home and think nothing more of it.

Ol girl was just gonna have to see me another time. I called her right after I found out that I would not make the flight, in my less than upbeat, energetic voice, I told her that I would not make this flight and, that I did not feel well enough to hang around at the airport all day to see how many other possible flights that I may not be able to get on. She seemed quite annoyed and unempathetic to how I was feeling. She just wanted to see me.

She tried to convince me without much success. I left that phone conversation with a bad taste in my mouth, but that was the least of my concerns. How the hell was I gonna gather the strength to go back in this weather and troop it all the way back home? I dared to wait for a ride share. They were backed up by several hours with this holiday rush of people trying to get around the city. Public transportation it is.

Once back at my residence, I had another problem that I had to tackle. Because I had not planned to be home, I had not gone out to do any grocery shopping. I would have to take that trip, but luckily I would drive. It was just as well, because this was starting to feel like a severe case of the flu. Because of my healthy lifestyle, it's rare that I get sick these days. Sure, a mild case of allergies once the seasons change, but nothing that would have me on my ass. I do not take medication, so this was going to be me against this virus.

I have my own nutritional supplement brand so I am always up on my *B. Rich Wellness multivitamins.* In fact, I have a *B.Rich Whey Protein Powder* shake first thing in the morning every morning, but the fact still remains, that I was sick and this was so out of character for me. I started to feel extremely hot and even to talk and have to make complete sentences was a chore.

My breathing was labored. I felt defeated. This felt like the flu, but it's older, bigger brother. Hmmm (hope you caught that)

I was bed ridden for two days, when I decided to go on my YouTube channel to make a video about being grateful for life. I was not feeling like this was the end, lol, I was feeling inspired to inspire others at that moment. I knew that I did not feel good, but if I could motivate others to feel good that it would fill my soul.

The video aired on December 26th, 2019 on my channel www.YouTube.com/brichscott In that video, I go on to say that I have not been this bothered by the flu in quite some time, in fact, it was many, many years. You can hear my voice laboring and hoarse. But I still managed to push through.

Right after that video a thought occurred to me. I carried a supplement called *Emergency Immune Booster w/ Elderberry & Cerebral- 300 CBD Gummies.* I immediately went to look at my inventory. YES! I had some available.. I don't know why I overlooked this, but I decided to go ahead and pop a few of those pills.

(The *Emergency Immune Booster w/ Elderberry* **bottle recommended 2 per day, I took 6!**

The *Cerebral- 300 CBD Gummies* said take **1, I took 3!-**

I DO NOT ADVISE THAT FOR ANYONE, BUT I HAD TO TRY A THING)

Normally, I would never do such a thing, and although I did not have any fear that I would not get better, because at the time, there was not a *FEAR* being narrated, in fact, nobody knew what this was at the time even though most people had and complained about this "Superbug"

I was more motivated to get well by being able to go ahead with my New Year's Eve plans more than anything else. And that would require me to not only be well, but to travel. Nevertheless, I had nothing but positive thoughts and the intention that I would be well soon.

You would think that I spoke life into the Universe, instead of it being the other way around.

In the next TWELVE HOURS, I felt better than I had in the last twelve days. I woke up the next day like my body had recovered from a hibernation of some sort.

Listen, by New Years Eve, I was in a Savannah club turning up!

In hindsight, me and my lady would have been better suited to stay in and enjoy some food, quiet company and some....well, you know. Instead we were out with these wild-ass college kids, which quite frankly, was not my cup of tea. We did not properly vet the venue where we needed to be. I would have preferred an environment more of our age and maturity.

Live and learn, right? But, my sickness was gone and that was that!

If only that is where the story ends, but it does not. We all know what happened in 2020, it started with Kobe's death and then it took a life of its own. I felt there was a change happening. The Universe had spoken to me and allowed me to hear and see some things that I was quite grateful for. The day after Kobe passed, I wrote a post on my Facebook page, saying how this is going to be the most different year you have ever experienced in life. And yes, that is easy to say every New Year, but I had already known that *this* year would be different.

February 2020

I was in Brazil enjoying the culture. Back in the US, before I left, there were reports of a deadly virus spreading across the Asian continents. I was planning a trip to Japan right after Brazil. Many said that would not happen because of this virus that was running wild. In my mind, I thought, "virus-smirus". Ain't no virus stopping me from traveling to where I want to be. In Brazil, there was not too much talk about any virus or bug, so I thought.

I didn't really understand Portuguese and I did not stay in the house long enough to watch any of the programming even if I did. I was there to run these streets! It wasn't until I was at the gym where I started to pay closer attention to this. I was on the elliptical, getting my last 10 minutes in, when I saw a TV screen that had the news on. I could not hear the TV, wouldn't understand it even if I did, but I saw the words *COVIDA-19* and from the looks of this report, people were not panicking, but were becoming concerned.

We originally had thought about staying in Brazil longer than we planned, but after we saw that report, my lady said that it may be in our best interest to depart at the time we established. *Scaredy-cat.* We got back to the US and I remember this very clearly, a week after being back home, the United States closed its borders for international travel. *Whoa!*

I have never heard of such foolishness in my lifetime. I still did not understand how this was even possible and what was the exact THING going on. It was not until maybe a few weeks later when the whole globe shutdown was when I put two and two together. Oh damn, I had this thing and so did MANY others prior to us knowing what it actually was called! Corona-virus. Covid-19, Kung Flu. Whatever you wish to label it

I can DEFINITELY go into all the conspiracy in this, but that will be for another time when a write the full book, ***UnF**K COVID.*** For now, I will stick to the facts regarding my personal situation and experiences. By midyear, many people were losing their minds and even scared to open a window to breathe in fresh air, including myself. They had me shook! I was spraying and wiping down every surface that I came into contact with bleach. I was afraid of a damn plastic bag because the virus lived on the surface for years they said (exaggerating) but you get the point.

There was a whole lot of misinformation, conflicting information, incorrect information...and this was being given out from WHO and the CDC. (Just an alley oop for my conspiracy theorists… *WHO*, and Owl...ok!)

Listen, I had the N95 mask, the respirator mask, and then when they said a damn scarf would do, I said "Oh, Hell nah", something wack is up! That is also around the time I figured out how and where I originally got in from, the first time.

It was in San Diego, California around December 16th, 2019. My ladies mother and sister had a cough and cold that had been lingering around for a while.

Didn't think anything of it. Why would I?

Fast-forward about a year later, they had got tested and they had the antigens for the C-Virus in their blood, which confirmed what I had already suspected. Yep! That was my original contraction. But that Emergency Immune Booster & CBD Gummies, seem to calm that stuff down with the quickness, but it was not until the second time around with this joker is where I knew, at least for me, that this is going to be my go-to, 1-2 punch!

March 2021

Atlanta is like a second home to me. And with that being said, Atlanta is now the Florida of the world. CRAZY AS FUCK!

During the whole time that most of the United States ...and the WORLD was on lockdown, Georgia, especially Atlanta, were one of the main places turning up and flexing about it. The states were reporting that the numbers were high and that death tolls were getting out of control. Again, funny that the CDC is in Atlanta, yet the numbers are out of control? Hmmm. Moving on, I was not fucking with ATL.... Sike!

It was the first time I had been in Atl since the travel restrictions were lifted; I was out and about enjoying the freedom. I was so surprised when I went into the gym to work out that many people were not wearing masks. This was my kind of place. It wasn't that I was not traveling; I was on a plane as soon as travel was allowed, towards the end of 2020, but I did not make my way to Atlanta until March 2021.

I had just left Las Vegas in January of this year and it was still kind of slow moving (was in Las Vegas in July...They back to full throttle for the most part)

So what did I do when I was in Atlanta? I did what most do. Had a ball and risked it all, lol..

Nah, but I was in this club called, Suite Lounge. I had a couple of my ladies with me and we were all in there with everyone else with no masks. There were strippers on the pole, people smoking weed, people all in one another's social distancing parameters.

Fuck a social distance! I was just on a goddamn plane, stupid!

I said to everyone with me, I know for facts, corona was all up in the club that night and we will for sure know in the next two weeks. So, don't be surprised when we are not feeling well.

But, weeks later, not even as much as a cough. Hmmm, maybe I still have the antibodies a year plus later from 2019, Cool!

May 2021

After being back in Boston for about a month, I needed to take care of some business regarding my nutritional supplement brand, which is actually based out of Atlanta. I had to take a tour of the facilities and make sure the operations were running smoothly. While out there, I had my ladies with me (three of my sister wives) , my daughter, my niece and my ex. We all went out to different events together and separately at different times.

My niece and one of my sister wives already resided in Atlanta, one of my sister wives lived in Savannah and took the drive down, and myself, live-in sister wife, and my daughter flew out from Boston. The ex lived in Atlanta as well.

The reason why this is so important is because, we were all in close quarters of each other many times within that week, but only 2 out of 7 of us got hit with the bug! Lucky me.

And if the other 5 *did* get the bug, they sure were anti symptomatic as fuck!

The second time that I caught this thing it was a bit more interesting.

My symptoms for the first three days were a slight headache, (that was a tell-tale sign for me, I don't get headaches) mild cough, and a low grade fever. I wasn't tripping though, as long as I could breathe, I was cooling. Plus I was still working out (not in public), When I was out I made sure to wear a mask, because I knew I was contagious and I did not want to accidently infect anyone. It was pretty much business as usual.. Until that 5th day!

Boom! Loss of taste and smell!

Now THIS sensation was HELLA WEIRD! Ya hear me!

It was like being trapped in your own body. There was a sense of claustrophobic paranoia associated with it. It was real trippy because I can breathe perfectly fine, but could not smell anything. The taste of food was absent from me. I learned real quickly to channel what I have taught others to do, and that was to go inside yourself and calm your mind. There is no way for anyone to understand this experience unless you actually go through it.

I immediately went back into my supplement bag, and used what I did the first time, but this time I tripled up! (Not advisable, I'm just saying what I did) My *B.Rich Wellness Emergency Immune Booster* & my *Cerebral-300 CBD gummies*. I added a few extra multivitamins this time.

I quickly got over being sick within five days, but my taste and smell returned exactly on day ten.

I definitely contribute my short time with Covid again to my supplements.

I have heard of numerous people whose smell and taste did not return for months. I am not sure if any products would help if someone has their smell & taste compromised for that long, but if you can attack it from the jump, perhaps supplementation will save some time in your recovery process.

Thanks for downloading!

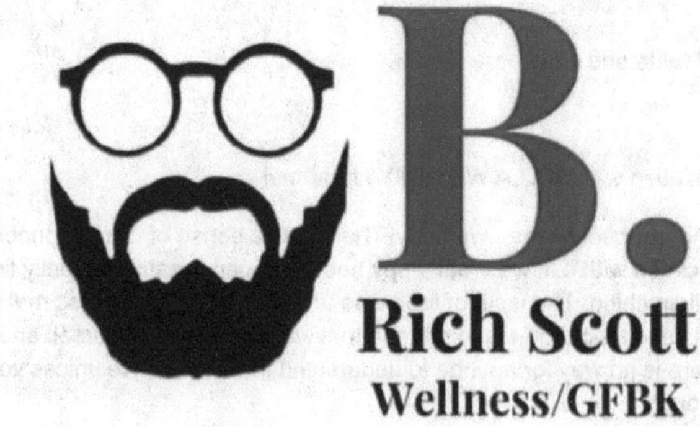
B.
Rich Scott
Wellness/GFBK

www.ingramcontent.com/pod-product-compliance
Lightning Source LLC
LaVergne TN
LVHW031113090826
845145LV00013BA/3025

9781737884057